BEAUTIFUL HAIR & HEALTHY SCALP SECRETS & REMEDIES

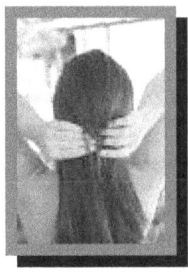

Mia Wadsworth, 2006

Download your bonuses here:

http://www.dryitchyscalpremedies.com/bonuses

CONTENTS

IMPORTANT

Please note that although the oils and remedies presented in this book are known to be the most gentle to sensitive skins and scalps - as with any natural substance some oils such as Thyme can in some individuals cause mild irritation on rare occasions and some oils should NOT be used at all while pregnant – It is recommended that as a precaution you should patch test all oils/formulas before application or addition to your shampoos.

Firstly, well done for starting the journey towards permanently getting rid of your itchy, dry or sore scalp and restoring your hair and scalp to its natural and beautiful condition.

For years I was painfully aware of how it feels to suffer from scalp issues. For personal reasons I wrote this e book and I have spent hundreds of hours compiling all that I am about to share with you. Discovering the secrets to having gorgeous hair and a healthy scalp every day of the rest of my life is now something I wish to share with you.

My desire is you too can share the benefits of what I now know so you too can be free of itchy flaky or dry scalp.

I am so excited to share with you all I have discovered in my quest to find natural solutions to relieve, cure and prevent these insidious problems from EVER coming back to haunt you.

So read on and enjoy – and once again thank you for taking the time and energy to buy this book – I am sure you will be very happy (and relieved!) you did.

Please let me know how you get on or ask any questions, I look forward to hearing from you.

Mia

We are all born with the potential to have a glorious head of hair. Our hair and scalp are supposed to be healthy in our natural state, but why is it that so many of us are suffering instead from itchy, flaky dry scalp and brittle lack-luster hair with straw like split ends, and sometimes even thinning patches? Not surprisingly, many people suffer self esteem issues when they suffer from hair and scalp problems.

The basic chemical make up of hair is keratin, a strong protein that also makes nails. Each strand of hair comes to the end of its natural life from between two and seven years when the hair is released from the follicle and new hair grows in its place. All of this cycle is going on without us even realizing it.

Beside each follicle there is a sebaceous gland which normally secretes sebum to lubricate our hair and naturally moisturize the scalp.

Theoretically we should all have beautiful hair and a healthy scalp all the time if we eat the right foods and watch what we put on our hair. If you eat plenty of fresh food, cut down on stimulants such as coffee tea, and alcohol, eat plenty of fresh veggies and fruit and a diet rich in cold pressed oils and unsaturated fatty acids, and get enough sleep, you theoretically shouldn't suffer from any dry scalp conditions.

However, we have been conditioned into treating our hair and scalp on an almost daily basis with a chemical cocktail. It is a medically recognized fact that our body absorbs significant amounts of what we put on our skin. In general we are not made aware by most hair and skin product manufacturers of ALL the ingredients they choose to use in their products. No wonder it is difficult to make an informed decision on hair care products when we can be so misinformed! Marketing experts are very clever telling us about the good stuff – i.e. "contains fruit oils" but obviously not so keen to tell us about the not so good stuff. Most of the time you'll find it's the other ingredients often in their cheapest form they add that can be silently doing damage to our scalp, hair, skin and eyes. YUK!

Even more unbelievable is the fact that some natural products contain synthetics which are dubious. Take, for example, Lauramide dea, part natural but also part synthetic, which is used to build up a lather and which is not only drying to the hair but can cause scalp itching and dermatitis.

A list of other hair and scalp nasties include:

- Oleyl betaine is a synthetic substance used to reduce static but it causes dandruff, dry hair and a dry scalp, and is toxic when absorbed through the skin.

- Other commonly used toxins are Sodium C 14-16 and Olefin sulfate, petroleum derivatives used as wetting agents.

- Other nasty ones are Sodium lauryl sulfate, Sodium beryl sulfate, and Sodium laureth sulphate (SLS). These can all cause a range of allergic reductions, hair loss, a dry flaky scalp, or skin rashes. Unfortunately these are often disguised with "natural names" but are actually toxic.

Not only are they damaging your hair, but also can be causing harm in other parts of your body. SLS's are also found in many liquid soaps, toothpastes and dishwashing liquids.

I'm sorry if this is leaving you with your mouth wide open but reading this e-book on dry, itchy scalp remedies will be a reality check to say the least. My aim is not to scare monger you with the facts but to inform and guide you towards the most natural solutions there are.

I found out what they were doing to my scalp and body the hard way. My best friend and I both suffered from terrible itchy weeping scalps for years – the mystery as to why we had this condition (and symptoms) had only deepened after using various different dandruff shampoos and other drug store medications trying to fix the problem. For both of us seeking advice about dry, itchy scalp problems was proving to be exhausting and producing very little results.

It was embarrassing going to the hair salon and having my hairdresser ask if I had head lice or some nervous itch problem. I developed a severe reaction to drug store or supermarket hair dyes and colorants (thank heaven for the natural hair-dyes I have found now). And I dreaded anyone running their hands through my hair – even my husband (a sort of dandruff and scab phobia).

I was at my wit's end, sick of continuous itching and sore scalp hell. I'd had enough and out of the frustration in not having found a solution, I cautiously threw away all the products I had spent hundreds of dollars on – the medicated shampoos, lotions and potions. Believe me at the time I thought I was being brave but I think it was more shear determination to find a cure. I knew everything else wasn't working so what else did I have to lose?

It was then that I decided to go back to nature in the hope of finding some answers.

Not just how, but why?

One thing I did know was that this was a "modern day problem" so there must be an answer hidden in history. If these problems only just began in the modern times, but not in the past, then the past must have had something right.

As luck would have it, I was given a shampoo to try (Neways shampoo, www.neways.com) which was derived from natural surfactants (more on this later). I used this shampoo for 2 weeks and my itching COMPLETELY disappeared. I could not believe it. HOW COULD IT BE THAT SIMPLE? So I gave some to my friend who had been suffering from the same complaint – same result. She had a perfectly healthy scalp and hair two weeks later. I found out (after researching and testing this breakthrough on others with this problem) that we were not the only ones and that this is a VERY common thing. I also discovered soothing natural remedies for fast relief.

After investigating and applying what I knew, for the first time in years I noticed my hair growing thicker and much healthier from the nourishment I had been giving my scalp instead of stripping it and soaking it in irritants and growth retardants. I had people commenting on how shiny and healthy my hair was after having dull dry brittle "straw like" hair before. My hair and scalp felt conditioned, healthy and vibrant with NO weepy sores or any itching whatsoever.

It felt so good having solved my own (and my friends') dilemma that I was inspired to share this information with others who were also suffering unnecessarily from a "scalp crisis." So I did - including helping my friends' father who had suffered from severe psoriasis for 18 years. We made some very simple basic changes and his psoriasis cleared up almost completely. Word spread that we knew something about this problem and interestingly many friends, and friends of friends, then other people wanted to know where they could get some of this shampoo too because they were such great results.

Wow. This REALLY is fantastic I thought. However, despite having cured myself and seeing so many others with results, I confess to being one of those people that feels the need to test everything (in order to eliminate all doubt), so after 8 months I decided to really put this theory to the test. I went to a good hair salon and bought an expensive off the shelf shampoo (moisturizing for dry hair formula). And the itching was back after one week of using this shampoo.

Eureka, I thought. The shampoo is DEFENITELY the culprit and it confirmed what I had concluded—that the cause MUST lie IN the shampoos I had been using. This lead me to spend a long period of time researching this 'phenomenon' and conducting research on ingredients in beauty and hair products.

I was one of the lucky ones not to have developed more severe conditions such as eczema or psoriasis. Later I will explain what I discovered through research as to why these conditions evolve, and what else you can do to get rid of them. We also used this knowledge to completely cure our two-year-old's chronic eczema.

What I discovered SHOCKED ME but I was also RELIEVED to have finally found the answer. It was very simple and made sense.

What I discovered and applied inspired me to share my experience and educate other victims of this frustrating problem, to lighten the weight of their frustration and discomfort with a simple solution so they do not have to go through the pain of having to waste hundreds of dollars with no results or answers like I did.

Let's start by first covering some of the common "scalp complaints" that you may be dealing with, and then I will share with you the underlying cause of almost all scalp conditions, they can be traced back to a simple source.

WHAT ARE COMMON SCALP CONDITIONS?

Common doesn't mean dry, itchy scalp is not incredibly irritating. Common just means there are a lot of people suffering with the same thing.

If you want to get to the root of your problems, so to speak, you need to be able to identify what your problem actually is. Of course, many scalp conditions will look alike, so going to your doctor may be the best way to get an accurate answer.

Just remember what may not look much to others, means the difference between a good day or a bad one.

RED BURNING ITCHY SCALP

Red burning itchy scalp can be characterized as any tingling, burning, prickly, and sensitive to the touch or a fiery hot sensation. Often associated with an allergy, sunburn, chemical burn (sensitization of the scalp), or fungal infection.

DANDRUFF

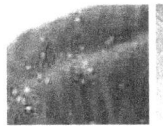

Dandruff as most of us know is the process of continual shedding of skin cells on our scalps. Often the cause of dandruff is simply the result of toxins, pollutants and products that have built up on the scalp particularly products like silicone – a cheap commonly used artificial shine enhancer in conditioners many of which are found on supermarket shelves.

When the natural balance of our scalps is disturbed, this creates the perfect environment for the yeast fungus Melassezia Globbosa to move in and thrive. This is when the natural process of shedding our cells gets a little out of hand resulting in an unsightly condition known as "Seborrhoeic Dermatitis" (fancy name for dandruff) and we see the highly visible tell-tale signs of flaking and crusting.

Did you know – It is thought that about half the human population suffers from dandruff and that men tend to be more susceptible? (BBC News report November 2007)

If you have an itch scratch it – right?

The accompanying itch and urge to scratch are often made worse by the multiplication of the fungal yeast pityrosporum-ovale (having one big party on your scalp). Another follow on effect of this is that the relentless scratching by the sufferer can cause small lesions which weep and ooze or become infected. How incredibly cruel and nastily ironic is that just by merely having a dry itchy scalp will then cause even more problems? Please at this point do not give up! – there are remedies that will cure this condition. I just need to share some important information with you first.

Lumps bumps and sores are also common when the scalp is highly irritated or sensitivity has been aggravated. Candida can be an underlying cause of yeast infections of the scalp.

RINGWORM

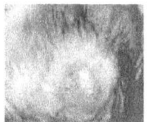

Ringworm of the scalp (tinea capitis) is a superficial fungal infection of the scalp. Scalp ringworm is caused by mold-like fungi called dermatophytes. Ringworm infection occurs when a particular type of fungus grows and multiplies anywhere on your skin, scalp, or nails. It is far more common in children and symptoms include red, itchy patches on the scalp, leaving bald areas. The skin might itch and be red and peel or be scaly, have swollen blisters or a rash (that can spread) and looks like black dots. The rash is highly contagious. It is normally treated with over the counter products containing miconazole, clotrimazole, or similar.

Sometimes prescription antifungal skin medications, such as ketoconazole are needed to clear it up. There are also products direct from nature's factories that can aid the healing process and act as natural antibiotics, although it must be said that ringworm is an aggressive fungus which needs to be monitored closely and treated accordingly.

DRY SCALP

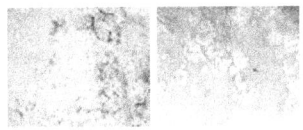

Dry scalp can feel "tight", a sensation that is sometimes accompanied by flakiness. It is often the result of natural oils being stripped from our scalps by the frequent use of shampoos, hair dyes and or other hair products.

SCALP DERMATITIS

Dermatitis of the scalp (Seborrheic dermatitis) is an inflammatory disorder affecting areas of the head and body where sebaceous glands are most prominent. It can vary from mild dandruff to dense flakey and greasy scale. Once again it is often an accumulation of toxins and products built up on our scalps that our body is trying to rid itself of.

ECZEMA OF THE SCALP

Eczema of the scalp similar in appearance to Seborrheic dermatitis but instead has the name Atopic dermatitis.

SCALP PSORIASIS

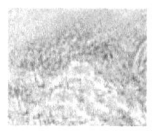

Scalp Psoriasis commonly occurs on the back of the head however multiple areas of the scalp or the whole scalp may be affected. Scalp psoriasis is characterized by thick silvery white scales on patches of very red skin and can extend slightly beyond the hairline. Scalp psoriasis, despite being partially hidden by the hair is often a source of social embarrassment due to flaking of the scale and severe 'dandruff'. Scalp psoriasis may be extremely itchy or on occasion have no itch symptoms. It can also cause temporary baldness on the affected areas. It is a common, chronic, inflammatory skin disease and is associated with increased risk of melanoma, squamous cell carcinoma, and basal cell carcinoma.

A survey recently done in the UK has some astounding key results and the one that screams out to me is 83% of people with psoriasis (includes all psoriasis sufferers) are dissatisfied with their current treatment! So it goes to show there are a lot of people out there just like you who have not only experienced the emotional and physical damage but have spent an awful lot of money on treatments that aren't working.

FOLLICULITIS

Folliculitis of the scalp is a superficial bacterial infection of the hair follicles. It is characterized by pustules around the hair follicles and symptoms include painful brushing of hair and tenderness when rubbing your scalp around the hair follicle sites. Treating with antibiotics for the particular bacteria is the usual course of action but can eventually cause restistance to the antibiotic used. Options include applying Evoclin Foam which is topical. Folliculitis is commonly caused by staph bacteria which also reside inside the nose and sinus cavity. Natural oils such as tea tree and lavender have good antibacterial properties and can also be used to treat this condition.

STRESS RELATED ITCHING

Stress can contribute to or worsen scalp itching as it plays havoc with our immune system and hormones which have an effect on production of sebum from your sebaceous glands. Although it can contribute to the problem it is still somewhat of a myth. It may appear that you have a "stress rash", but it is more likely that the problem was already there in a less noticeable way, then aggravated by increased stress levels making it harder for your body to deal with the problem on its own and eliminate the problem.   Many of the treatments below include stress relieving properties – like Lavender oil for example which calms the mind and soothes the body.

Did you know Lavender has been around for over 2500 years? Wow, the Egyptians first used it in the mummification process, the romans used it in for cooking and bathing and even King Charles V1 France slept on lavender filled pillows!

HAIR LOSS

There are quite a few different factors that can cause hair loss from many common shampoo ingredients, damaging hair follicles and inhibiting hair growth - to increased levels hormones like DHT – testosterone in men. Stress can also be a factor for women suffering from alopecia. Thankfully there are solutions - some drug based and some are naturally derived like

Revivogen. Natural oils such as lavender have also been found in studies to stimulate and repair follicles resulting in thicker hair.

Most people aren't aware of the damage from common shampoo ingredients which also inhibit new hair growth. They also don't know that they can use powerful natural remedies with similar properties to commercial products to help counteract the causes of hair loss and at the same time encourage & stimulate hair re-growth, improving the health of your scalp, follicles at the same time.

In my opinion, the reason most people grab what they think is the solution off the supermarket or chemist shelf is for a number of reasons. One could be the millions of dollars these producers can spend on advertising. We are a trusting bunch us humans and we tend to believe the glossy, expensive advertising.

Note most of the natural ingredients I mention are easily sourced or grown for a fraction of the cost – incredible really isn't it.

Secondly in my opinion the other big contributor is it is far easier to buy something within reach than it is to hunt it out. It is only natural, but most people who suffer unnecessarily with a dry and itchy scalp will eventually find their way to a perfect natural cure that suits them.

What helped me find a cure for my own dry itchy scalp condition was to look at the various causes of this problem. From simple allergies caused by shampoo ingredients to liver dysfunction I completely understand how overwhelming this journey can be. With marketers out there trying to sell products to "apply" and "rinse with" we tend to overlook what is causing this scalp condition in the first place. To illustrate this point, Anthony Robbins tells the story of the doctor and the people that needed help:

One day, as he's walking by a stream, a doctor hears someone yell "Help. Help. Someone is drowning."

Most people would walk past and get some help. Some would freeze, not knowing what to do. Not a doctor. A doctor would jump right in, drag them out, perform CPR, pump the fluids out, and do mouth-to-mouth resuscitation and hopefully revive the person.

But as soon as the doctor is done, guess what he hears coming from the river? TWO yells going "Help." So he jumps in saves them both, and then he hears 4 more yells. 8 more yells.

In fact, the doctor is so busy saving people that he never has time to go upstream to see who's throwing them all into the water.

This is a predicament many people are in when trying to solve scalp and skin problems. Wouldn't it make sense rather than just blindly throw money away on various TEMPORARY solutions to treat the symptoms (which if incorrectly prescribed may make the problem worse & harder to treat PROPERLY) before you even know why you have the condition in the first place.

If you understand the CAUSE you can SOLVE the problem PERMANENTLY instead of perpetuating the problem by treating the symptom with a "band-aid" approach.

In our modern society there are so many opportunities for our bodies to fall out of balance, especially with the wide use of medications and antibiotics combined with the huge amount of milk and bread we consume. This is resulting in an overabundance of yeast and fungal infections particularly of the dermis (skin). We have become a time strapped society, running from one thing to the next. The message is to slow down and have the time to address our own health issues because we are worth it.

Yeasts (like Melassezia Globbosa) are able to multiply and flourish. Then when our bodies are already "out of whack" and our scalps are raw, burning, itching and flaking, we go out and apply MORE unbalancing and aggravating products to our already tender sensitive scalps. This seems to just mask the problem without getting to the root cause.

Did you know that shampoos are among the most frequently reported products to the FDA? (Federal Drug Administration of the USA) Why?

Shampoos contain ingredients (such as foaming agents) which are very effective in cleaning the hair and scalp and allowing you to enjoy that "lots of suds fresh and a clean feeling."

While this is fantastic for stripping your hair of unwanted dirt and grease, these same commonly used ingredients (in over 90% of shampoos) are also very effective in stripping skin cells and your scalps' natural oils resulting in a dry scalp, flaky skin and itchy tender scalp.

The FDA reports include eye irritation, scalp irritation, tangled hair, swelling of the hands, face and arms and split and fuzzy hair. Some of these ingredients are even used for testing by drug companies to intentionally cause a reaction on a subject's skin so they can test their "anti-inflammatory" products on them.

So what are these nasty ingredients that are allowed in our everyday shampoos? Two of the main offenders are Lauryl Sulfate (SLS) and its close relative Sodium Laureth Sulfate (SLES). These two ingredients are commonly used in many soaps, shampoos, detergents, toothpastes and other products that we expect to "foam up." Just look on your dish detergent or shampoo bottle label to find them.

Obviously, both chemicals are very effective foaming agents, chemically known as surfactants.

The sodium lauryl sulfate found in our soaps is exactly the same as you would find in a car wash or even a garage, where it is used to degrease car engines. Interesting thought isn't it? The last time I looked my body is made up of a completely different element than my motor car!

In the same way as it dissolves the grease on car engines, sodium lauryl sulfate also dissolves the oils on your skin, which causes a drying effect. It is also well documented that it denatures skin proteins, which causes not only irritation, but also allows environmental contaminants easier access to the lower, sensitive layers of the skin. It also corrodes the hair follicle and impedes hair growth. This effect has been blamed for many cases of premature hair loss and it takes hair longer to grow when it has been affected by SLS. How about we think about our hair and scalp the way we would our flower or vegetable garden. Would you put something on your garden that would, in some cases, harm the flowers or even kill them? I am still shocked that a chemical used in car degreasing process is included in shampoos.

But perhaps most worryingly, SLS is also absorbed into the body from skin application. Once it has been absorbed, one of the main effects of sodium lauryl sulfate is to mimic the activity of the hormone Estrogen. This has many health implications and may be responsible for a variety of health problems from PMS and menopausal symptoms to dropping male fertility (effects fertility of male fetuses) and increasing female cancers such as breast cancer, where estrogen levels are known to be involved. In our great grandparents day they used more natural products to clean their hair and I bet the cancer rate wasn't nearly so high. It's not all doom and gloom though we are lucky in the modern world to have access to information so at least we have the choice on what to use to clean our hair and scalp. What we do with this information is really up to us.

Now imagine going to a day spa for a luxurious pampering session, you lie back to enjoy the therapist cleansing away oils and gently steaming open your fresh pores so they are ready and open to readily soak up all of the beneficial ingredients and nutrients into your awaiting thirsty skin. The beautician pours on a potent elixir of ... antifreeze or engine degreaser which is quickly absorbed into your open pores into your body – that's not exactly what you signed up for, is it? But that's what we do in the shower daily with the chemicals in our bath products. Wouldn't you rather be nourishing not polluting our delicate skin and our cells in our bodies?

Is it any surprise our scalps cry out to us burning and itching with dermatitis and flaky scalp or melassezia globbosa sometimes leading to scalp eczema, psoriasis?

At best, these SLS's are classified as only "mild skin irritants" (according to the scientific community relatively safe as long as rinsed off skin immediately after use). Is it any wonder your eyes sting if the suds make their way into your eyes ouch? And if you think this sounds nice, did you know they add anesthetic to baby "no more tears" shampoo so your children cannot feel the pain of the sting from these ingredients damaging their delicate eye membranes – absolutely remarkable isn't is.

So why is a dangerous chemical like this used in our soaps and shampoos?

The answer is simple - it is cheap.

Years ago scientists believed that the skin was a barrier to the environment that did not absorb substances that came in contact with it, and so did not comprehend the possible negative impact of ingredients in shampoos and other personal products on our bodies. Of course we now know this is not the case. So being fully aware of the facts, why didn't the shampoo manufacturers change their ingredients?

Alternatives to these chemical agents (although readily available) are not dirt cheap like their toxic counterparts. So if you were a multi-national conglomerate selling millions of bottles of shampoo to pre-conditioned customers, who had been buying your products for generations and were blind to the dangers lurking in their bathrooms - would you bother to make changes? Probably not - unless you were morally driven as opposed to fiscally motivated? Just remember we are talking big money and big business here. Once again we have access to this information if only we look in the right places, so congratulations on finding this e-book and reading it.

In 2004 the University of Bath's Department of Chemical Engineering in England were granted 95,000 pounds to carry out new research to look at compounds from seed oil and sugar and how they could replace these petroleum based products used in cleaners and shampoos with the aim of making them more eco friendly. The fact that petroleum products are not completely biodegradable and therefore do not entirely break down in our environment means as global citizens we should look to change our old habits.

It is fantastic news that such research programmes are being run and looking at ways in being more eco friendly. What we should so is shift our mind set to anything that is being researched as being more eco friendly is probably friendly to our own physical body as well.

And is it any coincidence that many of the same conglomerates make a fortune from selling anti-dandruff treatments and other medicated shampoos for scalp conditions all over the world? It's interesting to me that the same products we buy to treat itchy scalp also contain the very ingredients that created the problem in the first place.

Increased awareness, a healthy lifestyle, holistic treatments, prevention, and natural remedies mean bad business for the drug companies. In fact, the healthier you get, the less money the medico-pharmaceutical industry makes considering that 90% of pharmaceutical sales are from "maintenance" drugs. They keep you coming back to buy medicines that treat the symptom and not cure the "disease" itself. Sounds like the biggest scam ever doesn't it?   My goodness to think about how vulnerable we all are about different products really takes your breath away.

Advertising is very clever and there is a real psychology around it. In Supermarkets around the world manufacturers pay extra for certain positions that will entice those hungry shoppers to buy more of their product. Chocolates and sweets of all varieties are placed at checkouts and in positions that taunt the young and old just to pick and buy. This doesn't all just happen by accident, teams of people work on ways to get us to buy more of their product. It once again comes down to making money.

It is much the same with hair products. Conditioned by advertising (drug companies and shampoo manufacturers) that skin/scalp conditions are diseases that just show up, for no apparent reason, and that the only solution is their products – (which of course we will need to keep buying and using to keep the problem at bay) we buy more of their shampoos. I mean, we consumers don't know what's causing all of these ailments so isn't it fantastic to have all these drug researchers doing all of this work so they can produce the right information and products to solve our problems?

And the poor doctors are only doing their best for us too with what they know.   Just think about who primarily educates them about new advances in medicine - the pharmaceutical companies' sales people.

So how do we know what these contaminants are and what are they called?

I have listed below for you ingredients to look out for but first a word on Sensitizers and Irritants; they are not the same so here is a rundown on the difference:

SENSITIZERS, IRRITANTS & INGREDIENTS USED IN PRODUCTS

SENSITIZERS

Sensitivity is the result of a response by our immune system from being exposed to a substance or "foreign body" that it wants to keep out of the body. Sensitivity develops over several years (or months in children).

The reason sensitizing chemicals often "slip under the radar" is because the first use of a sensitizer (e.g. from a synthetic colorant in hair dye) may not trigger a reaction, but subsequent or repeated use can cause a person to develop an allergic reaction to even very low levels of the original or related substance. A reaction can "hit you" seemingly suddenly, when really it is the result of a "build-up" of your immune system's response over a period of time.

Your body is an intelligent organism, in the sense it knows what is good for you and what isn't and this "signal" from our own body is telling us something. We really need to listen better!

Irritants on the other hand are quite different to sensitizers and allergens which involve the immune system. An irritant is a non-allergic inflammatory reaction at the site of where the substance was applied (yes sensitizers can cause rashes elsewhere on the body). The difference is that dermatitis (a non fungal dandruff) is commonly the result of irritation directly from a product, whereas allergens and sensitizers (especially the highly sensitizing products used in hair dyes and colorants and henna tattoos) will effect your immune system in a way that is difficult to "get at" because once you develop a sensitivity, it's with you forever.

What are these ingredients called then? Below I have listed the culprits in most shampoos and some conditioners.

Formaldehyde: Many companies put formaldehyde in their shampoos? It is not only an inexpensive preservative and disinfectant; it is also a suspected cancer-causing toxin. Even the sound of this toxin makes your skin crawl, literally.

Coal Tar: Many kinds of shampoo designed to treat dandruff and flaky scalp contain coal tar, but you will not find it on any product list of ingredients. It is disguised with names FD & C or D & C color. It has been found to cause potentially severe allergic reactions, asthma attacks, headaches, nausea, fatigue, nervousness, lack of concentration and cancer. Shampoo companies really need to be far more transparent about EVERY ingredient they are so cleverly trying to hide.

SLS's Sodium Laureth and Sodium Lauryl Sulphates: SLS's are foaming, degreasing detergents also found in toothpastes, liquid soaps, dish wash liquid, engine degreasers and car wash etc. Exposure to SLS can lead to a burning sensation, coughing, wheezing, laryngitis, shortness of breath, headache, nausea and vomiting, SLS penetrates your eyes, brain, liver and remains there long-term.

Being a cell mutagen, it degrades cell membranes because it can change the genetic information in your cells and damage your immune system and reproductive organs in male fetuses. It can cause blindness (scientific studies have proven that this compound damages protein formation in the eye tissue) and can lead to cataract formation. After damage to the eyes has been done, your eyes cannot heal properly because SLS retards the eye healing process. Also retards hair follicle growth making hair harder to grow. This is all difficult reading and probably by now, if you are anything like me, you may be feeling slightly abused.

Alkyl-phenol ethioxlades are chemicals in shampoos that have been proven to reduce sperm count.

Propylene glycol: is another ingredient you will find in most shampoos and conditioners and many moisturizers. It is not only ineffective, it is dangerous. Derived from petroleum products, it is commonly used in antifreeze, de-icers, latex, paint and laundry detergent. It can cause irritation of nasal and respiratory passages and if ingested, can cause nausea, vomiting and diarrhea.

Research also shows that it alters cell membranes and causes cardiac arrest. Carefully check for these dangerous chemicals on the labels of all your personal care products to save yourself from severe health problems.

EDTA (ethylene diamine (tetracetic acid) Is a stabilizer used in cosmetics to prevent ingredients in a given formula from binding with trace elements that can exist in water and other ingredients; the technical term for this function is a chelating agent. It can cause: dizziness, drowsiness, headache, cloudy film in eye, otitis media, plugged ears, watery eyes, cough, nasal congestion, rhinorrhea, sore throat, arrhythmias, nausea, vomiting, abdominal cramps, anorexia, diarrhea, elevated liver function tests, hemorrhoidal symptoms, metallic taste.

D&C Green 5 A coloring agent used in cosmetics which can cause irritation to skin, mucous membrane and eyes.

Selenium sulfide used in antidandruff shampoos which can cause irritation to skin, mucous membrane and eyes. How cruelly ironic that an ingredient that is supposed to help your dry itchy scalp is adding to it?

Salicylic acid Treats acne by causing skin cells to slough off more readily, preventing pores from clogging up. This effect on skin cells also makes salicylic acid an active ingredient in several shampoos meant to treat dandruff. Salicylic acid is toxic if ingested in large quantities, but in small quantities is used as a food preservative and antiseptic in toothpaste. The carboxyl group (−COOH) can react with alcohols, forming several useful esters. The ester with methanol is methyl salicylate, also known by the name oil of wintergreen (sounds like it is organic isn't it which we know its not). The hydroxyl group (−OH) can be acetylated to form acetylsalicylic acid (aspirin). Salicylic acid can also trap oxygen (O2) and initiate free radical reactions. Also known as Beta Hydroxy Acid (compare to AHA), salicylic acid is the key additive in many skin-care products for the treatment of acne, psoriasis, calluses, corns, keratosis pilaris and warts. Use of straight salicylic solution may cause hyper pigmentation on unpretreated skin for those with darker skin types. Salycylic acid does occur naturally in Willow Bark so a treatment containing willow bark can be beneficial.

Ketoconazole is a synthetic antifungal drug used to prevent and treat skin and fungal infections, especially in immunocompromised patients such as those with AIDS. Due to its side-effect profile, it has been superseded by newer antifungals, such as fluconazole and itraconazole. Ketoconazole is sold commercially as an anti-dandruff shampoo.

Itraconazole is a triazole antifungal agent that is prescribed to patients with fungal infections. The drug may be given orally or intravenously. Itraconazole is a relatively well tolerated drug (although not as well tolerated as fluconazole or voriconazole) and the range of adverse effects it produces is similar to the other azole antifungals.

Possible Side effects:

- Elevated alanine aminotransferase levels is found in 4% of people taking itraconazole

- Congestive Heart Failure

- The cyclodextrin that is used to make the syrup preparation can cause diarrhoea.

- Contact your doctor if the following side effects are present as they may indicate a greater problem.

- nausea, vomiting, abdominal pain, fatigue, loss of appetite, yellow skin (jaundice), yellow eyes, itching, dark urine, pale stool

Voriconazole is a triazole antifungal medication used to treat serious fungal infections. It is used to treat invasive fungal infections that are generally seen in patients who are immunocompromised. These infections include invasive candidiasis and aspergillosis.

Common side effects include: Blurred vision, increased eye sensitivity to light, or other visual changes, Nausea, vomiting, or diarrhea, Headache, Swelling or water retention.

Rare but life-threatening side effects include: Severe liver damage, Allergic reactions to the medication

There are numerous drug interactions and the advice of a pharmacist should always be sought.

Can you see a pattern emerging here? We know with most drugs there are side effects but we really are not aware of the seriousness that these common shampoo ingredients can cause.

It sounds strange and perhaps a little hard hitting I know but it is like a doctor giving a drug addict a nice bag of drugs and saying there you go help yourself, knowing full well they will be back once all the drugs have gone asking for more. It just doesn't fix the problem, and in most cases is actually adding to the problem.

Calcipotriol (INN) or calcipotriene (USAN) is a topical medication used for the treatment of psoriasis. Calcipotriol has minimal side effects apart from skin irritation and can be used over the short- or long-term, and achieves results quickly. It is available as a cream, ointment, or solution. It is also available in combination with betamethasone.

When you understand the physical and mental impact of psoriasis like some of you may do, it is absolutely crucial that there is a natural and sustainable cure. Even an ingredient or product that has a mild side effect just doesn't hit the mark in my opinion.

Sulphates: To function well, all shampoos and body washes require a cleansing agent to degrease the skin and hair. There are four main groups of cleansing agents (surfactants) comprising sulphates, soaps, sulfonates and carboxylates.

Many surfactants are derived from petroleum, although some are naturally derived but produced with a little help from the petroleum industry. For example, Olefin Sulfonate can be derived from petroleum or coconut oil. If you take a look at the label of most shampoos, shower gels, bubble baths and hand washes, you are likely to find sulphates featuring high in the list of ingredients. Sulphates are strong, cheap cleansing agents preferred by the cosmetic industry. The most common being sodium lauryl sulphate, sodium laureth sulphate and ammonium lauryl sulphate.

Sulphates can be highly irritating and there are question marks over their long term safety. Of all the sulphates, Sodium Lauryl sulphate (SLS) has had the worst press. This strong detergent is used in skin care products including shampoos, liquid hand washes, shower gels, bubble baths and toothpastes. Considered safe in small doses, although found to be a skin and eye irritant in higher concentrations, this chemical has again been linked with many health scares, including cataracts, skin rashes, hair loss, flaking skin and mouth ulceration ("The effect of two toothpaste detergents on the frequency of recurrent aphthous ulcers," a study by Herlofson BB and Barkvoll P, Acta Odontol Scand. 1996 Jun; Department of Oral Surgery and Oral Medicine, Dental Faculty, University of Oslo, Norway).

SLS has also been linked to nitrosamines formation. Nitrosamines are recognized carcinogens, which can be formed when two otherwise safe chemicals, nitrous acid and amines are combined. Nitrosamine production can occur from a reaction from these chemicals during the processing stage of a product or during storage. SLS can become contaminated with other chemicals during processing, including chemicals such as triethanolamine (TEA), diethanolamine (DEA), monothanolamine (MEA) which are common ingredients in shampoos. This resulting reaction between such chemicals can result in nitrosamine production.

DEA, MEA, TEA DEA, MEA and TEA are used as solvents, emulsifiers and detergents. They have been found to cause allergic reactions, irritate the eyes and respiratory tract (Rev Environ Contam Toxicol, 1997; 149: 1-86), and dry the hair and skin. Studies have also shown that they may be carcinogenic, especially to the kidneys and liver (J Am Coll Toxicol, 1983; 2: 183- 235 and Rev Environ Contam Toxicol, 1997; 149: 1-86).

Luckily there are many natural surfactants available with lots of beneficial moisturizing and cleansing properties. Coconut and yucca are two examples of natural cleansers that are just as good at cleaning your hair and scalp as SLS if not better.

Yukka plants are just so easy to grow and require very little maintenance. Why is it the alternative makes more sense with no side effects, proving to be even cheaper than these toxic ingredients and yet we are bombarded with all these nasties?

Petrochemicals: "The risks of synthetic chemicals extend beyond human health. Many of the ingredients in cosmetics are environmental pollutants. Along with the waste produced during the manufacturing process, millions of gallons of synthetic chemicals are washed down the drain and into sewers everyday. Petrochemicals commonly used in makeup, skin creams, and hair care products not only contaminate our waterways but also can destroy marine life". (Excerpt from "Drop Dead Gorgeous" by Kim Erickson).

The main lubricants in many moisturizers, conditioners and hand creams are liquid paraffin, propylene glycol and mineral oil. These by-products of the petroleum industry are used in large numbers of cosmetics and toiletries due to the fact that they are very cheap. These petrochemicals can cause photosensitivity (i.e. can promote sun damage), and strip the natural oils from the skin causing chapping and dryness. They can also prevent the effective elimination of toxins from the skin, resulting in acne and other disorders.

These so called beauty products are used by millions of people around the world, who have no idea what damage these ingredients have the potential to cause. Because they are promoted in such an alluring way, with beautiful models in exotic settings we are all guilty of wanting to look and feel the way the advertisement plants in our conscience.

Propylene glycol is a common ingredient in moisturizers, yet also used extensively in brake fluids and antifreeze products. This ingredient can result in sensitivity reactions and is the most widely used moisture-carrying ingredient in cosmetics. This ingredient has been found to be a neurotoxin by the National Institute for Occupational Safety and Health (the Medical Post, 27 September 1994) and it has recently been connected to contact dermatitis, kidney damage and liver abnormalities (Page 28, Drop Dead Gorgeous).

PEG or polyethylene glycol, and its immediate family of PEG-6, PEG-150 and other similar ingredients: These chemicals are commonly found on cosmetic and personal care product labels as surfactants, cleansing agents, emulsifiers, skin conditioners, and humectants. Dangers have been highlighted by recent research, regarding impurities found in various PEG compounds.

Research published in The International Journal of Toxicology by the cosmetic industry's own Cosmetic Ingredient Review (CIR) committee, found impurities found in various PEG compounds including ethylene oxide; 1,4-dioxane; polycyclic aromatic compounds; and heavy metals such as lead, iron, cobalt, nickel, cadmium, and arsenic.

Perhaps most troubling of these findings is that PEG compounds are routinely contaminated with the carcinogen 1,4-dioxane. Studies show that 1,4-dioxane readily penetrates human skin. According to the National Toxicology Program in its Ninth Annual Report on Carcinogens, "1,4-dioxane is reasonably anticipated to be a human carcinogen." In experimental studies, 1,4-dioxane increased incidence of liver and lung tumors and carcinomas of the gallbladder.

"The Environmental Protection Agency considers 1,4-dioxane a probable human carcinogen, based of the "induction of nasal cavity and liver carcinomas in multiple strains of rats, liver carcinomas in mice, and gall bladder carcinomas in guinea pigs" (EPA, 2003).

In 2002 the FDA expressed continuing concerns about 1,4-dioxane, noting its potential to contaminate a wide range of products, its ready penetration through the skin, and the evidence linking it to systemic cancer in a skin painting study (FDA 2000).

A consumer could identify products with potential 1,4-dioxane contamination by scanning product labels for the common ethoxylated surfactants that may contain the impurity, which according to FDA are identifiable by the prefix, or by the designations, of 'PEG,' 'Polyethylene,' 'Polyethylene glycol' 'Polyoxyethylene,' '–eth–,' or '–oxynol–' (FDA, 2000)."   (www.ewg.org/reports/skindeep/report/impurities.php Parabens/Synthetic   Preservatives).

Parabens: Parabens are preservatives which are found in the vast majority of cosmetic and skin care products. Preservatives by their very nature are designed to kill living organisms. According to Pat Thomas in the "Ecologist March 2006", "Widespread concern about the use of cosmetic preservatives stems from the fact that human skin is comprised of living cells, and so preservatives, even if they are used in small quantities, present a risk to the integrity of the skin and, should they be absorbed into the bloodstream, to the rest of the body." Take the time and have a think about it for a minute, is anything that is designed to extend somethings shelf life good for you? Nature doesn't work that way, something has a shelf life – fruit for example, and then it doesn't. That is why nutritionists will always tell us fresh is best. If you have ever had the joy of growing your own vegetables then you would have experienced the shear pleasure of really tasting how vegetables should taste. It is one of the best experiences in the world – you can literally taste the goodness and the freshness.

Parabens are added to kill bacteria and inhibit mold, but they have been found to mimic oestrogen (see E Routledge et al "Some Alkyl Hydroxy Benzoate Preservatives (Parabens)are Estrogenic", Toxicology and Applied Pharmacology 153 (1998):12-19), and having also been found in breast cancer tumors, there are understandably growing concerns regarding their safety.

Parabens are known as skin and eye irritants, and have also been linked to damage to sperm production, due to their hormone disrupting nature. Some manufacturers argue that they are used in such small concentrations that they cannot have any adverse effect on humans. I'm not sure that is enough of an argument myself, how about if we think of a court of law for any crime that is committed – sorry Your Honor I only burgled him a little bit – that sounds ridiculous doesn't it?

However, as they cannot be broken down, the concern is that over time they can accumulate in the body. "Endocrine disruptors are chemicals that interfere with the normal functioning of the body's hormones by either blocking the body's natural estrogen or acting like an estrogen impostor…

While natural estrogens are vital to normal human development, synthetic hormone disruptors have been linked to a reduction in sperm, impaired thyroid function, breast cancer, and even behavioral problems such as attention deficit hyperactivity disorder (ADHD)" (from "Drop Dead Gorgeous" by Kim Erickson).

A recent report has suggested a worrying potential threat to the developing fetus and young babies, finding that butylparaben and proplyparaben can have an adverse effect on the reproductive system of young male mammals. The study concluded that the preservatives 'adversely affect the secretion of testosterone and the function of the male reproductive system': Oishi, S, "The effects of butylparaben on the male reproductive system in mice", Arch Toxicol, 2002 and Oishi, S,

"Effects of promptly paraben on the mail reproductive system in rats", Toxicol Ind Health, 2001.

Fluoride: Fluoride is a common ingredient in most toothpaste. Included for its dental benefits in tackling tooth decay, it is also said to be an acute toxin with a poison rating higher than lead. It has been linked to health problems such as brittle bones, osteoporosis and (incredibly) porous dental enamel. In hypersensitive people fluoride also causes eczema, gastric distress, headaches and weakness and has been linked to genetic damage, including cancer, and hyperactivity and attention deficit disorder in children.

Ever thought about why water filters are so popular at home and in the workplace? It is because we are now expecting to have better quality water to drink without unwanted ingredients, just look at the huge amounts of bottled water now available to the public to buy. Synthetic Fragrance: Synthetic fragrances can result in many unwelcome symptoms including headaches, dizziness, allergic rashes, skin discoloration, violent coughing and vomiting, and skin irritation. Clinical observations has shown that synthetic fragrances can affect the central nervous system, causing depression, hyperactivity, irritability, inability to cope, and other behavioral changes. The majority of allergic reactions to skin care products can be traced to artificial fragrances.

Imidazolidinyl urea and DMDM hydantoin: These formaldehyde-forming preservatives can cause joint pain, allergies, depression, headaches, chest pain, chronic fatigue, dizziness, insomnia and asthma. There is some research that also suggests that they can weaken the immune system. These ingredients are found in skin, body and hair products, as well as antiperspirants and nail polish. (Source http://www.skinorganicsonline.com/index.php?main_page=product_info &products_id=128)

HAIR DYES

Common hair dyes contain some of the most carcinogenic and sensitizing ingredients of all. If you have ever had a "fake tattoo" that is henna based, then beware – there have been many cases of severe allergic reactions to the compound PPD (phenylenediamine) requiring hospitalization in people who have applied a hair dye (black or dark brown in particular) after having had a henna tattoo.

See http://www.hennaforhair.com/ppd/ppdreaction/medarticles.html for an example.

There are also many more cases of reactions that have occurred from sensitivity to compounds in hair dyes. In rare cases scalp reattachments have been necessary after the scalp opened up due to the swelling.

A woman with a mild adverse reaction to hair dye:

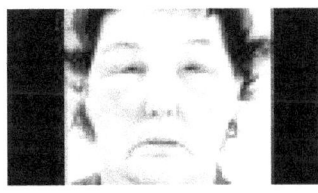

The main ingredient found to be highly sensitizing (and can cause blindness) is phenylenediamine. Other irritating ingredients are hydrogen peroxide and ammonia. You will discover that THE MAJORITY of off the shelf and even gentler salon dyes include one or more of these ingredients.

Salon brands such as Keune are generally less harsh on your scalp and hair so if you must, use them.

I would go to a salon and advise asking for a "sensitive scalp" hair dye. There are many brands which are NOT harmful and leave your hair in much healthier condition due to their gentler active ingredients and conditioning properties. I have listed some on the next page.

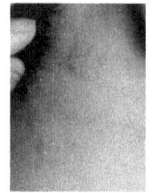 If you have ever applied a hair dye to your head and felt a "hot" or "prickly" sensation, then this could be a sign of a sensitivity developing. Another sign is if you have red patches around the periphery of your hairline and on your scalp itself (see photo) then this can also be an indication of sensitizing. If you find that dandruff shampoos have irritated your skin (or even some brands of plain shampoos) then this is yet another "red flag" warning sign.

I myself have burned my scalp after using a supermarket brand hair dye – my reaction appeared to come "out of the blue" but had I known what the warning signs were preceding this, I could have seen it coming.

I had never had a history of skin issues as a child and had used hair dyes before without a problem. However, the last time I had used this particular brand dye prior to this event, I had noticed that my scalp had felt "hot and tingly" which was a new thing for me. I had also noticed that smell was particularly "intense" to my senses which was another sign to be aware of - this is another one of nature's ways of warning us.

Thankfully, I took action immediately and rinsed the dye out. This helped but I still needed to swallow an antihistamine tablet to calm the irritation down. I was lucky not to have had an even more severe reaction.

Here is a list of hair dyes that are mild to your scalp followed by natural remedies that with time will color your hair when used on a regular basis:

- Clairol Loving Care Color Lotion

- Igora Botanic

- Logona Henna

- Rainbow Research Henna

- Salon Formula Sun In

- Naturstyle Hair Colors

- Clairol Light Effects

Any Henna based dyes are fine (providing they contain no chemicals such as phylenediamine as well of course). Henna is a natural dye which thickens hair (coats it) as well while coloring your hair safely. Note again that some people who have used henna tattoos have had a severe reaction to phenylenediamines after having used henna tattoos).

Below are some natural gentle hair rinses that have been used for centuries to color and condition hair:

- Chamomile is a highly beneficial and conditioning as a natural dye for light hair and ground black walnut husks soaked in water then strained - the liquid applied and left on is good for darker hair.

- Another remedy is to use about half a cup each of rosemary and sage leaves which have been simmered in water until it reduces down to a concentrated "stew". Strain and apply to your follicles combing down to your ends. When applied daily this will cover grey hairs and restore hair to a brown color.

Dry scalp is usually a symptom of a lack of oils on your scalp which have been stripped away by the harsh detergents in your shampoos. Normally a dry scalp will return to its naturally moisturized condition with the use of a good quality non-stripping shampoo such as those I recommend without the need for any other treatment. You can use oils like coconut also (more on this later).

I know these days no-one can imagine not washing your hair but for one reason or another, probably due to being ill we haven't been able to. More than likely you have then had oily hair and for most people this happens very quickly. Shampoo is taking natural oils out of your hair and whilst we may not go to such drastic measures we would survive not washing our hair and we would most likely be surprised at the results. If you suffer badly from a dry, itchy scalp it may be worth at least trying or minimizing the amount of times you shampoo your hair.

Scalp dermatitis (dandruff/flaking scalp or Melassezia globbosa) also is usually the result of a disturbance to your PH balance from harsh ingredients or from your body reacting to and trying to shed toxins, pollutants and products that have built up on the scalp. Adding to this problem, the stripping of the sebum in your skin creates a disturbance in the natural balance of your scalp thus creating an environment where bacteria/fungus can thrive.

Unfortunately most dandruff shampoos never address the cause of dandruff and deal with it. If you allow your skin to return to it's natural state, and use products that cleanse, detoxify and nourish but not strip your skin, allowing the natural pH and balance to return then your body will heal itself and return to a healthy state. It is also important to consider Candida as a cause of many recurring scalp infections that can also appear elsewhere on the body.

CANDIDA

Candida is a whole body yeast "infection" which can be caused by the effect of antibiotics removing the "good" bacteria in your bowel allowing the "bad" bacteria to thrive. Candida is worsened and further perpetuated by too much alcohol or bread consumption.

Candida is a genus of yeasts. Clinically, the most significant member of the genus is Candida albicans, which can cause numerous infections (called candidiasis or thrush) in humans and other animals, especially in immunocompromised patients. This results in itchy, and dandruff flakes or rawness/burning.

Another possibility is that you have simply dry scales or cracking on your scalp this can be the result of drinking too much milk and you may be suffering from lactose intolerance.

You can use the remedies listed later on in this book to soothe and rebalance your scalp.

Now for the shampoo residue issue - you can assist your scalp to cleanse itself & remove these pollutants by using a detoxifying shampoo, one containing zinc pyrithione or simply add a teaspoon of Rosemary oil to your shampoo which will help restore the natural balance to your scalp.

You can also use some of the remedies I list later on in this e-book such as those containing Manuka or Tea Tree oil. I also find lemon juice fantastic for removing build up – Juice of one lemon added to approx 2 tablespoons of conditioner. Mix together well and apply to wet hair, from the scalp and combing through to the ends of your hair.

Doesn't it feel great to get through a lot of scary and sometimes revolting information which helps you address findings and then make recommendations on your journey towards a cure?

Just have a look at some of these natural remedies I am recommending – there is a key point of difference between what my more natural cheaper options cost versus the cost of shampoos and conditioners that aren't so good for you.

RING WORM

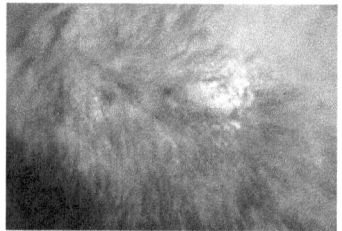

Ringworm, also known as Tinea, is a contagious fungal infection of the skin. Contrary to its name, ringworm is not caused by a worm and is NOT caused by shampoos (although they can increase the severity of symptoms). It is instead a highly contagious and aggressive fungal infection which if left untreated can spread to other parts of the body and cause unsightly circular rashes and localized hair loss.

In the case of ringworm, I would suggest you see a doctor for the appropriate treatment as it needs to be monitored closely and treated accordingly with the right medication.

What you can do though is to use Tea Tree oil and other antibacterial shampoos in this eBook to help soothe and inhibit its growth. While using a specified anti-fungal cream to clear it up, as well as the walnut recipe I have included in the remedies section, you can begin the healing process. We have all heard of the health benefits of omega 3 and walnuts are one of these natural products that contain this amazing element. Now walnuts can be spoken of as a healing food and not just a brain food! And that is what we are trying to do together here, we are trying to heal something so you don't continue to suffer with a dry, itchy scalp.

The best known sign of ringworm in people is the appearance of one or more red raised itchy patches with defined edges, not unlike the herald rash of Pityriasis rosea. These patches are often lighter in the center, taking on the appearance of a ring. If the infected area involves the scalp or beard area, then bald patches may become evident. The affected area may become itchy for periods of time. If the nails are affected, they may thicken, discolor, and finally crumble and fall off.

A Note On Conditioners: Many conditioners contain cheap shine enhancers such as silicone which can build up on your hair and scalp leaving your hair looking dull as do styling products. This can cause your scalp to flake and itch – or as we know it, dandruff. To remove it you need to use a clarifying shampoo prior to conditioning.

And by the way yes that is silicone I mentioned, the same silicone that is used in yep you guessed it breast enhancers! Not only breast enhancers but also commonly used in lubricants and adhesives. Unreal isn't it – personally I cannot see how these conditioners were even developed – how did we go from using silicones for glue to one day wake up and think we can now put that into hair conditioners and then sell it to people?

Use conditioners that will not artificially coat your hair with silicone but instead nourish your hair with moisturizing natural ingredients. See clarifying remedy for shampoo buildup later in this ebook.

As stated before, recent research indicates that "psoriasis is likely a disorder of the immune system. This system includes a type of white blood cell, called a T cell that normally helps protect the body against infection and disease.

Scientists now think that, in psoriasis, an abnormal immune system causes activity by T cells in the skin. These T cells trigger the inflammation and excessive skin cell reproduction seen in people with psoriasis" (Source: excerpt from Psoriasis: NWHIC).

Science tells us that both eczema and psoriasis are triggered by an immune response. Research also shows that psoriasis sufferers commonly suffer from acute liver toxicity /dysfunction as do some eczema patients. We know already that SLS's and other harmful chemicals are readily absorbed into our bodies via our pores and deposited long term in our liver. So how does this relate to psoriasis?

Well there are many theories and cases suggesting that if you detox your liver and "clear out toxins" that you can eliminate psoriasis. Stepping into your "common sense corner" for a moment, what do you suspect happens when your liver is so full of toxins that it can no longer deal with all the build up from foreign substances being absorbed into the body - then you add yet more of these toxins via your scalp/skin? It makes sense that your immune defense system will do whatever it can to get rid of them and keep them out. Once again our body is an absolute miracle, it is reacting to something that shouldn't be there.

So is it any surprise then that studies has found "scaling and flaking is the result of the body's immune system attempting to shed damaged or irritated skin to expel anything it identifies as unhealthy for its cells"?

There are some fantastic highly recommended psoriasis treatments out there such as Dr. Robert E. Connelly's book "Psoriasis Can Be Cured". He instructs his patients to follow a very strict program including diet, supplements and regular self tests to determine improvements in liver weakness.

I must say that Dr. Connelly has had some phenomenal results with his patients. Another fantastic cleanse specifically targeting psoriasis is sold by "Malcolm Harker". He offers a very good cleanse system and topical creams that are very beneficial (for other areas of the body) too. (Listed at the bottom of this e-book are some excellent creams, oil blends to assist in detoxification and other products that will give you relief as well as powerful natural remedies you can create yourself). But my favorite detox is "The Ultimate Cleanse" by The Herbalist. This in my experience is the best detox around.

Sadly a lot of people will try and tell you that detoxification and natural remedies are all rubbish but I wonder how many of them have actually tried to fix things the natural way? It just makes sense that what goes in or on our bodies affects it – not really rocket science is it?

This powerful cleansing program has been inspired by the great pioneers in the herbal cleansing field – Dr. Bernard Jensen, Dr. Richard Anderson and Dr. Sandra Cabot, along with traditional American Indian herbal cleansing. It is not the cheapest herbal cleanse on the market, but it is 100% effective. No shortcuts have been taken to save cost. Yet it is well priced for what it does. Similar herbal cleanse systems overseas typically cost three times as much.

The Ultimate Cleanse is a full intestinal, organ and tissue cleansing program which is completed over five or ten days. It leaves you feeling fresh, revitalized, light and clear (also with a clear head, skin and clarity of thought).

It has been formulated from a traditional herbal combination, which forms a unique process of detoxification involving the entire body. This method has been passed on by American Indians and has been developed to suit the modern lifestyle.

Common results include: Bowel activity improves, Toxic problems such as skin disorders, mucus congestion, fatigue, headaches (particularly migraines), arthritis, acne, obesity, addictions and asthma may all be reduced. It can help relieve gout, allergies, rashes, bowel disorders, indigestion, sinus, bloating, gas, hemorrhoids, blood pressure and cholesterol, parasite infestations, kidney and gall bladder dysfunction, peptic ulcers, Crohn's or diverticulitis and many other common complaints.

We have an average of 4-6kg in weight loss achieved and in some cases up to 20kg. The list of results depend on what level of cleanse your body needs to feel great.

All these health disorders have responded to the ULTIMATE CLEANSE:

- Acne

- Indigestion

- Allergies

- Intestine problems

- Arthritis

- Irritable bowel

- Asthma

- Kidney problems

- Bad breath

- Lazy Bowel

- Bloated feeling
- Listlessness
- Liver problems
- Boils
- Low energy
- Bowel problems
- Memory loss
- Candida
- Mucus congestion
- Constipation
- Obesity
- Depression
- Edema
- Digestive problems
- Parasites
- Eczema
- Psoriasis
- Fatigue
- Sinusitis
- Gas

- Skin & scalp problems

- Gout

- Toxemia

- Headaches

- Weight gain

- Heartburn

These methods are fantastic to help clean the liver so your body is not overloaded and does not manifest psoriasis or other conditions in order to protect itself.

Cleaning out your liver is important and is very effective in clearing up what you already have and feels fantastic - for a while. But where is the sense in going through this process if only to prepare our liver again for the next lot of irritants, carcinogens and formaldehydes we force into our bodies via our open receptive pores in the shower every day.

Even worse, the moisture, heat and cleansers we use, also remove our natural oil mantle thus causing further irritation (itchiness and discomfort) to our already tender sensitive scalps and ravaged hair follicles.

By now it should be fairly obvious that we need to take some steps to change the products we use and prevent starting the process all over again.

(Important note: I would highly recommend that if you suffer from psoriasis, that you do a liver cleanse.

TIP: While detoxing, it is important to refrain from eating pork, dairy as well as a high consumption of gluten based products. The main consideration to remember is to look for a program that is designed to move toxins out of your liver. Milk thistle is fantastic to help you cleanse as well as Cranberry juice.

PSORIASIS DIET DO'S AND DON'TS WHILE DETOXING

FOODS THAT ARE BENEFICIAL TO EAT WHILE DOING A LIVER DETOX ARE:	FOODS THAT YOU CAN EAT MODERATELY (MAKE UP TO ONE TENTH OF YOUR DIET) ARE:
Cranberries/Unsweetened Cranberry Juice	Apples
Dried Apricots	Beets
Fish	Blackberries
Green and other herbal teas	Blueberries
Herbs and Supplements	Carrots
High protein meats EXCEPT Pork including luncheon or baloney or sausage meat	Cherries
	Figs
High Sulfur Content Foods	Fresh Apricots
Low acid foods (too much acid contributes to liver toxification)	Black tea and coffee

FOODS THAT YOU CAN EAT VERY SMALL AMOUNTS OF WHILE DETOXING ARE:	FOODS THAT YOU SHOULD NEVER EAT WHILE DOING A LIVER DETOX TO ELIMINATE PSORIASIS
Artichokes	Alcohol.
Asparagus	All Beans
Avocado	Anything with a high sugar content or high yeast content or dairy products.
Beet Greens	
Broccoli	
Brussel Sprouts	Apples
Cabbage	Bananas
Cauliflower	Bottom Dwelling Seafood
Celery	Fresh Figs
Coffee and Black Tea	Grape Juice
Cucumber	High Sugar Foods
Dairy	Hominy
Eggplant	Huckleberries
Endive	Lentils
Honey Dew Melon	Macaroni
Kohlrabi	Mandarins
	Nuts

Leeks	Pears
Lettuce	Pineapple
Mushrooms	Pineapple Juice
Muskmelon	Plums
Peppers	Pork including luncheon or bologna or sausage meat
Radishes	
Rhubarb	Prunes & Plums
Sauerkraut	Raspberries
Spinach	Rice
Strawberries	Sweet Cherries
String Beans	Tangerines
Summer Squash	Tinned Corn
Swiss Chard	Tinned Succotash
Tomato Juice	
Tomatoes	
Water Cress	
Watermelon	

I have the utmost respect and admiration for people who proactively go about finding out everything they can do to keep healthy. It takes time and energy to do the self help style of healing a condition such as dandruff but sometimes that is exactly what we have to do – help ourselves! That means help ourselves as greedily as we can to look at the natural ways we can cure our dry, itchy scalp conditions, and that can go for any other conditions we may suffer from.

The benefits of self help is that we immediately know what is working and what is providing a cure. Within a very short time frame people start to feel the benefit as well as see the benefit. It is incredibly empowering and enables sufferers to stop being the victim and start being back in control. This shift in the balance of power will drive people towards absolute success. Once you start you won't be able to stop!

Now you understand some of the causes and what to avoid as far of the 'nasties' out there to look out for. (If you want a very comprehensive list of ingredients in shampoos and other products from food to toilet cleaners that have been rated for safety and which brands to buy or avoid – a good book to invest in is authored by David Steinman and Dr. Samuel Epstein titled "The Safe Shopper's Bible: A Consumer's Guide to Nontoxic Household Products".

This is a fantastic book covering non-toxic household goods from food to cosmetics. I will cover some good alternatives for you in this book also so it's easy to make changes and treat yourself to non toxic, nourishing products and remedies.)

Obviously the natural approach is best and avoiding using the harsh detergent-based shampoos is the surest way to combat scalp irritations.

Unfortunately it can be very difficult to know from looking at the labels which chemicals are actually in the products because they are disguised with 'natural' sounding names and some chemicals are naturally derived, but because they have been processed can contain contaminants and have become toxic through processing.

So I have listed below many alternatives to give you choices. In this way you can be sure of what you are putting on your hair, and save yourself a great deal of money at the same time.

YEAST AND CANDIDA SOLUTIONS FOR STUBBORN DANDRUFF AND ITCHING (IF YOU DON'T SEE RESULTS WITHIN THE FIRST WEEK)

As I alluded to previously, Candida, or an over flourishing of the wrong kinds of biotics, can be problematic by making dandruff and itching hard to get rid of, particularly if you have been on any antibiotics. The introduction of acidophilus and bifidus yoghurt cultures in yoghurt help to re populate your digestive tract with good bacteria. You can also take these in tablet form.

Here's what you can do: Yeasts love sugar, more yeast obviously and acidic foods, knowing that, you need to consider the following.

If you want to "pull out the big guns on Candida and yeast" and greatly improve your success, you should focus on what foods aggravate your condition to address the internal aspects of yeast infections.

As mentioned above, a good detox is highly recommended. If you cannot afford a detox, or do not wish to go through the process of a detox, avoiding or reducing your intake of certain foods it will make a big difference to the speed with which you can eliminate the problem. You can follow these guidelines for 2 to four weeks while going through the "healing and rebalancing" process in conjunction with treating your scalp with the natural remedies I have included for you.

BASIC ADVICE FOR TREATMENT

- Eliminate yeast bread from your diet for a couple of weeks. This sounds hard to do BUT it's actually not so bad if you replace sandwiches with wraps which are very delicious when you add fillings like Cajun chicken etc. Also tacos and burritos etc are good replacements for bread. Just stay off bread for at least 2 weeks and then just slowly re-introduce bread to your diet. Some people find they feel so good after this they never go back to eating the amount (of bread) they used to when you have discovered such delicious alternatives to eat instead. Shelly Young has a book Back To The House Of Health2 with lots of delicious recipes that are low or no sugar and super alkalizing. (Available from Amazon).

When we suffer with bad nutrition so does our hair. Dry, lifeless hair can be direct result from a bad diet. We live in a generation where obesity is at an all time high, fast food restaurants are actually increasing their profit and this is all during one of the worst recessions on record. There is no used blaming the take away industry – we have to admit that sometimes we are just too lazy to get off our buts and do something about it. Generation Y are said to be the ones who want it now and won't wait – we are all a bit guilty of that one I am afraid not just Gen Y's

- Eliminate or reduce wine, and beer, sugar and vinegar in your diet for the same period of time. This is like a mini detox in itself and will do wonders.

- The other thing to do is to eat raw (not cooked) almonds if you like them of course. Green leafy veggies are very alkaline so get stuck into salads if you like them and stir fry's. Meat is very acid as is coffee to try to lower your consumption of those a little (just watch what you eat but don't be too hard on yourself).

Omega 3's found in oily fish is great for skin and hair care. If you don't like the taste then omega 3 tablets are widely available. Making a few lifestyle changes will benefit you overall wellbeing both mentally and physically.

- Drink lots of water and drop a squeeze of lemon juice – or orange juice into your water bottle to alkalize your body each day.

- What you are doing by eliminating these for a week or two is starving the yeast and by eating yoghurt (or tablets containing acidophilus and bifidus) you are re-introducing the good bacteria allowing it at an opportunity to rebalance your system. The stricter you can be with this the faster the correction can take place.

- Even if you aren't able to do this "religiously" you can still take steps to turn the balance back in your favor by being conscious of this. I find just being aware of this helps you to make choices and you may be surprised how much of the yeast loving foods you have been consuming and also how easy it is to reduce them also make choices that help your body regain balance.

When you have too much yeast in your system you can feel foggy headed, be lethargic, have strong smelling urine, wounds can take longer to heal and there are many more subtle symptoms that are not pleasant. Most people find that when try get this handled they have more energy, are sharper in perception, they sleep better plus many more benefits. So it's a great thing to do for yourself – your body will no longer have to be fighting the imbalance 24/7.

LIST THAT NATURAL THERAPISTS RECOMMEND TO AVOID TO ELIMINATE CANDIDA

- Sugar - It is best to eliminate all forms of refined sugar, as it feeds the yeast and encourages its growth. These foods include: white sugar, brown sugar, honey, maple syrup, corn syrup, maple sugar, molasses, date sugar, turbinado, raw sugar, demerrara, amisake, rice syrup, sorghum. Read labels carefully. The hidden sugars to watch for include: sucrose, fructose, maltose, lactose, glycogen, glucose, manitol, sorbitol, galactose, monosaccharides, polysaccharides.

- Fruit - Fruit contain natural sugars that support the growth of yeast. The following foods should be eliminated:

- Frozen, canned, and dried fruit

- All canned and frozen fruit juice

- Oranges and orange juice

- Melons, especially cantaloupe (rockmelon) - These fruit often contain mold.

- Yeast - Foods that contain yeast should be eliminated. These include: Baker's yeast, Brewer's yeast, Engevita, Torula, and any other nutritional yeast. Baked goods raised with yeast such as breads, rolls, crackers, bagels, pastries, and muffins should also be eliminated.

- Foods Containing Gluten - These include wheat, barley, and rye and includes products made with these ingredients such as wheat bread, rye bread, and pasta.

- Vinegar (taken orally) - Vinegar is made with a yeast culture. Foods that contain vinegar include: White vinegar, red wine vinegar, apple cider vinegar, balsamic vinegar, mayonnaise, commercial salad dressing, ketchup, Worcestershire sauce, steak sauce, BBQ sauce, shrimp sauce, soy sauce, mustard, pickles, pickled vegetables, green olives, relishes, horseradish, mincemeat, chili sauce.

- Mushrooms - Mushrooms are fungi. Eliminate all mushrooms.

- Peanuts, Peanut Butter, and Pistachios -- Peanuts, peanut butter, and pistachios often have high mold contamination and should be eliminated.

- Alcohol - Alcoholic beverages provide sugar that feeds the yeast and stresses other organs such as the liver. Eliminate all forms of alcohol, including red wine, white wine, beer, whiskey, brandy, gin, scotch, any fermented liquor, vodka, rum, and all liqueurs.

- Coffee, Black Tea, Cider, Root beer -- Coffee and black tea create an extra burden for the body's stress-coping mechanisms. Regular coffee, instant coffee, decaffeinated coffee, and all types of black tea (including "fruit flavored" black tea) should be eliminated.

- Cider, root beer, and other fermented beverages should be eliminated.

- Aged, Moldy and Processed Cheeses -- Roquefort and other aged, moldy or blue cheeses should be eliminated. Also eliminate processed cheese such as cheese slices, Velveeta, Cheese Whiz, cream cheese, cheese snacks, and Kraft dinner.

- Processed, Dried, Smoked, and Pickled Meats -- These include products such as smoked salmon, pickled herring, sausages, bacon, hot dogs, pastrami, bologna, sandwich meats, salami, corned beef, pickled tongue, and kielbasa. These products are processed and many contain unhealthy nitrates and nitrites, so they are not recommended for use at any time.

- Packaged, Processed, and Refined Foods -- Canned, bottled, packaged, boxed, and other processed foods usually contain yeast, refined sugar, refined flour, chemicals, preservatives, and coloring. They are not recommended at any time.

The good news is - it is not difficult for you to find and integrate products into your life without these sensitizing or irritating ingredients. It is easy and inexpensive to protect yourself and your children from developing sensitivities early. Our son no longer has eczema because we made a few simple changes.

Sometimes we have to take matters into our own hands and "self diagnose" what is going wrong. Because these problems are so common now there are many ways we can find out if we have any food allergies. From testing kits to your local clinic it is very simple and very easy to find out what your body cannot tolerate.

There are plenty of natural hair product alternatives readily available which often are no more expensive and frequently much less than the everyday products you have been using. After all, you will no longer be paying for the expensive advertising paid for by big companies to sell you big name products.

There are many 'purist' natural product manufacturers who refuse to add toxic ingredients and fillers to their products. They prefer to invest in quality pure ingredients instead of chemicals and huge advertising campaigns. Your healthy hair will be shiny, full of body and bounce if you are using them because your scalp will absorb these healthy ingredients including vitamins, minerals, and nutrients.

The main thing to remember when shopping for natural shampoos is that they contain natural foaming agents - used in place of soaps and harsh detergents (SLS's) which serve as the primary cleansing and sudsing agents:

Some natural foaming agents are:

- Yucca (Yucca shidigera)

- Shikakai extract (Acacia concinna)

- Soap Bark Tree (Quillaja saponaria Molina)

There are also some ingredients that are considered to be gentle cleansers which are relatively safe - some very conditioning.

Very mild and non-irritating to the eyes:

- Amphoteric-2

- Amphoteric-6

- Amphoteric-20

- Cocamide diethanolamide

- Cocamide monoethanolamide

- Cocamido betaine

- Cocamidopropyl betaine

- Lauramide diethanolamide

- Lauramide monoethanolamide

- Polysorbate 20

- Polysorbate 40

- Sodium lauraminopropianate

- Sorbitan laurate

- Sorbitan stearate

- Stearamide diethanolamide

- Stearamide monoethanalomide

Also very mild and with good conditioning properties:

- Cocoyl sarcosine

- Disodium oleamide sulfosuccinate

- Lauroyl sarcosine

- Potassium cocohydrolysed animal protein

- Sodium cocoyl sarcosinate

- Sodium lauryl isoethionate

- Sodium lauroyl sarcosinate

Look out for these warning labels on the back of shampoo or conditioner bottles (and need I state that's it's best to avoid products like this):

Keep an eye out for products that contain beneficial antioxidants and natural fragrances derived from natural oils and essences. There are many synthetic fragrances that cause irritation and so avoid products that are not naturally fragranced.

The reason I have gone into so much technical detail and given you the names of these ingredients is so you have the option of making informed buying decisions. You have the knowledge to know what you are buying when you come across a product you "like the look of." However, if you are like me, having to inspect every bottle of anything I buy is not the way I like to shop.

So to save yourself this inconvenience, there are a few simple things you can do to avoid this hassle:

The first thing you can do is to avoid buying supermarket or hair salon products UNLESS they specialize in organic or natural shampoos and hair dyes. I have tried finding "big brand" shampoos that do not contain SLS's – even baby shampoos – but found that very few supermarket stocked brands do not contain toxic ingredients.

There are some brand exceptions which I have listed at the bottom of this book. I have found that the higher end salon shampoos are more likely to have been tested for scalp sensitivities. Many still contain irritating ingredients like SLS's, but they are often not as concentrated and are less likely to react to your scalp because they generally contain more beneficial ingredients to nourish your hair.

The second thing you can do is to shop at a store that specializes in selling non-toxic products or a health store. Products need not cost more and in fact often are less than salon brands.

The third solution is to save yourself the time and hassle of finding these products yourself and benefit from my efforts in finding some fantastic brands that are very economical and highly effective. I have done the homework for you. Most of the natural shampoos I include in my "safe" list below are jam-packed with beneficial nourishing ingredients – and even the foaming agents such as coconut derived cleansers are also moisturizing and healing.

Below is a comprehensive list of my favorite brands of pure, economical, safe non-irritating products. They are all loaded with beneficial, pure and concentrated ingredients which have made an incredible difference to the condition of my hair and scalp. These companies offer shampoos, conditioners and body washes.

I have also listed a fantastic source for aromatherapy oils which are very effective in helping with ailments and for general wellbeing. I have also listed below some 'remedies' you can make yourself to use directly or as additives to add to your shampoo that naturally combat dandruff, eczema and fungal or bacterial infections of the scalp. Essential oils penetrate deeply into the hair shaft and follicle and produce healthy, shining hair. There are seven essential oils that encourage new hair growth also.

Many oils and other products listed are available in select health stores; however my personal preference is to buy them online. Here are some of the retailers I use:

PRODUCT RECOMMENDATIONS

See http://www.dryitchyscalpremedies.com/store for our own range of Soothing Scalp Remedy products.

You can also visit http://www.dryitchyscalpremedies.com/links.html for links to products listed in this ebook.

BE ESSENTIALS (NATURAL AROMATHERAPY PRODUCTS)

http://www.aroma.com.au/

Balanced Essentials supports a balanced approach to health and lifestyle as the key for a successful and happy existence.

Cheryl Gilbert is the owner/creator of Balanced Essentials and has a background in traditional medical care. With this in mind, Cheryl developed a range of aromatherapy blends, perfumes, incense and aftershave made from pure essential oils, which are energized using crystals. These products were created with the express purpose of enhancing awareness and activating self-healing.

They combine pure essential oils of the highest therapeutic quality. Each oil is subjected to quality control procedures to ensure scientific evidence of its properties. This unique collection of products, superbly presented, is created using blends of essential oils that describe the effect and are color coded to relate to an energy centre of the body. The inclusion of crystals to promote and amplify the properties of the products supports results that offer a profound and beneficial approach to health and wellbeing.

(BE Vital is excellent for application to lumps, bumps and itchy areas)

NATURALLY NGAROMA

http://www.naturallyngaroma.co.nz/

At Naturally NgaRoma, they strive to create the most natural of skin care and cosmetics we can without harsh cleansers. The soaps and skin care products are handmade in small batches to ensure freshness. Handmade soaps are cured for at least 5 weeks before being packaged for sale to you. This ensures the soap is super mild and extra luxurious. In addition to wonderful fresh, natural soap and skin care products, they have added a range of 100% natural mineral cosmetics. Mineral cosmetic are the most natural makeup a woman can wear. They not only make your skin look natural they can also improve the condition of your skin. They have no talc, no synthetic fillers or dyes and are free from petrochemicals and preservatives. This formulation is based on inert, naturally occurring minerals that are pulverized and blended to create a variety of products from foundation to eye shadow, eyeliner, blushes and lip color.

THE [A'KIN] RANGE (BY THE PURIST COMPANY)

http://www.puristusa.com/

Asia Pacific http://www.purist.com.au/

The (A'kin) difference lies in its uniquely high concentration of special nourishing and other active botanical ingredients - using only those scientifically proven to be of most benefit to the hair, skin and scalp. The result: naturally exquisitely fragranced, genuinely natural, ingredient-rich products for radiantly healthy skin and hair.

The Purist Pledge: "Each and every high quality, genuinely natural ingredient selected for [Alchemy] is present in an amount sufficient to have a significant positive effect, and is free from objectionable impurities and toxic preservatives." Will Evans Director of Research Founder - The Purist Company

- Shampoo: Most shampoos function from the action of one or two chemical cleansers and foam booster. These simple mixtures are too harsh, and consequently chemical coating agents (usually silica based) are added to counteract the stripping effect and to give the hair shine. [A'kin] takes a totally different approach. They use a synergistic complex of up to six special gentle cleansers, all derived from natural ingredients such as corn, sugar cane, palm and coconut oils and tapioca. Synthetic coating agents are not required and the hair and scalp are left naturally clean and in perfect condition to adsorb the deeply penetrating nourishing ingredients from state of the art "skin friendly" conditioners.

- Skincare: [A'kins]'s uniquely pure skincare formulations are rapidly absorbed, delivering natural nutrients deep into the skin, without the risk of irritation or allergy. Enjoy the luxury of [Alchemy]'s ingredient-rich products as they nourish and nurture your skin, while the delicate aromatherapy fragrances relax your body and sooth your soul.

OJON NUT OIL RESTORATIVE TREATMENT

http://www.ojonhaircare.com/products/OJT0001

Highly concentrated pure Ojon Nut Oil, it instantly hydrates and rebuilds distressed hair, leaving it extraordinarily soft, shiny and healthy looking. This is ideal for hair that is damaged, dry, dull or chemically treated. And these products provide essential conditioning for ALL HAIR TYPES, even if your hair is already in good condition.

SULFUR

Sulfur is very beneficial for scalp conditions, and rumor has it that it is also good for stimulating hair growth. Applied topically to the skin, sulfur-rich creams are very successful in clearing up scalp conditions, particularly in treating Seborrhoeic Dermatitis. Sulfur creams have been shown to reduce the increased sebum production, while ridding the scalp of itchy scales.

Sulfur rich foods you can supplement your diet with include: eggs, seafood, beef, veal, tongue, liver, chicken, dried apricots and peaches, cabbage, Brazil nuts, peanuts and cheddar cheese. Onions, garlic and leeks are also rich in Sulfur.

SOME OTHER SPECIFIC 'SAFE' SHAMPOO BRANDS THAT CONTAIN LOW OR NO IRRITANTS

You can also visit our store http://www.dryitchyscalpremedies.com/store for our own Soothing Scalp Products

- Aveda www.aveda.com

- Neways www.neways.com

- Mukti Botanicals

- Aubrey Organic Hair Products www.aubrey-organics.com

- Bindi Hair Wash

- Earth Science

- Faith In Nature www.faithinnature.co.uk

- Miessence   www.miessence.com

- Head Pure and Basic Lite Shampoo

- Natural Instinct   www.naturalinstinct.co.nz

- Ivory

- Jhirmack Lite

- Legona www.legona.com

- Mera

- Naturalbodycare   www.naturalbodycare-nz.com

- Paul Penders www.paulpenders.com

- Thursday Plantation www.thursdayplantation.com

- Desert Essence Tea Tree Oil Shampoo www.desertessence.com

- Urtekram

- Ecco Bella

- Putting It Right Store products www.puttingitright.com

- Hemp seed shampoos (such as Richmond Nature brand available from health stores). Hemp is known to be very beneficial for clearing up skin irritations & soothing itching - particularly beneficial for psoriasis sufferers

- Hemp shampoos available from your local health store or online, you can also add beneficial healing oils - particularly good for psoriasis and eczema.

ITCHY SCALP REMEDIES AND SHAMPOOS (FOR RELIEF WHILE STILL ITCHING)

IMPORTANT NOTE: Below these recipes I have included in some other uses for these oils so you get the best value from purchasing them even after you have treated your scalp and hair. You can also visit our store http://www.dryitchyscalpremedies.com/store for our own Soothing Scalp Products

Neem and Tea Tree Fungal Fighter

This is must have formula for dandruff. The oils needed are low cost and have many other uses after you have eliminated your dandruff.

Add 10 drops of Neem oil and 10 drops of tea tree oil to 2 tablespoons of vegetable or nut oil (e.g virgin coconut, jojoba, sweet almond, safflower, sunflower or olive oil).

Apply thoroughly to your scalp covering the whole scalp area. Massage in - it feels great - refreshingly tingly and very soothing. Leave on your scalp for a minimum of 10 minutes and overnight if you can. Shampoo as normal, with non-toxic shampoo, of course.

Do this two to three times over a 10 day period and you will notice the dandruff will disappear fast.

This mixture is a highly effective dandruff fungal and bacteria fighting remedy. It's also good for ringworm and scalp infections like scalp acne. (Neem is quite a strong smelling oil - if you find it too overpowering or if you want extra conditioning and healing you can add 10 drops of Lavender oil).

These oils are good to keep in your cupboard to treat cuts, acne bites and Neem will kill insects so it's good for head lice as well.

OTHER NATURAL ANTI-BACTERIAL AND ANTI-FUNGAL DANDRUFF REMEDIES

GO TO http://www.dryitchyscalpremedies.com/remedy_calculator.html to create your own personal remedy suited to YOUR hair & scalp issues:

Manuka oil (tea-tree or Melaleuka alternifolia) is has good antibacterial, antifungal, and anti-inflammatory properties providing an effective natural medication to control the symptoms of Seborrheic Dermatitis. Add 10 drops to your favorite shampoo. It is always best to patch test diluted Tea Tree first as it is a strong oil.

UMF Active Manuka Honey (available from health stores) has been considered a remedy for many health conditions since ancient times. Active Manuka Honey is unique to New Zealand and contains non-peroxide antibacterial agents which can inhibit the growth of certain bacteria that cause slow healing wounds such as eczema and burns. The higher the rating the better e.g. UMF 18 is better than UMF 16 or 12. Apply to wounds or sores for healing.

Lucas's Paw Paw (Papaya) Ointment This ointment is very calming applied to eczema rashes to help with itching. Note: Paw Paw is not anti-bacterial.

Chamomile For Inflammation And Conditioning: Chamomile is a flower that is renowned for its cosmetic and conditioning benefits to skin and hair. It makes a great conditioner for hair and also enhances color in blond and red hair. Wash your face with chamomile tea a few times a week to add a glow to your skin.

Chamomile is also good to use as a compress for inflammation and chamomile oil dabbed on scalp sores is very soothing.

Chamomile tea is readily available from the tea section of your supermarket or you can make your own by boiling a pint of water and adding 2 teaspoons of chamomile flowers. Rub into scalp after straining.

Dandruff Formula 1: 18 drops Rosemary oil, 10 drops Thyme oil, 8 drops Sage oil.

A variation of this if you have these herbs in your garden (and don't want to use oils) is to add 1 Tablespoon each of these chopped fresh herbs from your garden and steep them in boiling water (e.g. in a teapot).

Allow the mixture to cool to luke warm, strain the herbs out. Then saturate your scalp with the solution and leave on for a minimum of 10 minutes then rinse (or leave in if you wish).

Dandruff Formula 2: 1 Tablespoon Honey, 5 drops Thyme oil, 5 drops of Eucalyptus or Peppermint oil, 3 drops Sage oil and 5 drops Carrot oil. (You may substitute the oils for freshly chopped herbs steeped in water if you wish). Good for scalp odors too.

Healthy Scalp and Shiny Hair Formula: 10 drops Sage oil, 10 drops Lemon oil, (or tsp lemon or lime juice), 5 drops basil, 15 drops of Eucalyptus or peppermint oil

Soothing Scalp Formula: Mix ½ teaspoon active manuka honey with 5 drops of Chamomile and 5 drops of Lavender Oils then add to ½ cup of chamomile or sage tea. Saturate scalp with this mixture, and leave for 10mins then rinse in the shower.

Super Simple Dandruff Formula: Add 20 drops of Manuka (Melaleuka alternifolia or Tea Tree) oil to your shampoo and/or 5 drops of Eucalyptus oil. This is highly stimulating to your scalp also.

Dry Scalp Itch Formula: Mix together Rosemary and Sage oils with Tea Tree, Ylang Ylang, and Atlas Cedarwood (equal quantities) in distilled water. Sprayed directly onto the scalp to soothe itchiness and is very moisturizing to the scalp as well.

Scalp Moisture Boost Formula: 20 drops Neem OR Jojoba OR Evening Primrose. Add 5 drops Lavender, Bergamot, Sandalwood or Chamomile to the base oil, mix with 3 Tablespoons of water and spray or dab on then massage into your scalp.

Lavender Oil: Burns and scalds, itchy bites and as an insect repellent, as a calming sleep aid added to the bath or moisturizer/vaporizer, headaches, cramps, convulsions and even fainting. The oil is antiseptic and anti-bacterial, and can be applied directly to burns and stings, where it will cool the pain. It will stimulate blood flow to the affected area, which may aid healing. The oil is analgesic (pain-lessening); rub it into painful joints for relief from arthritis symptoms, or into muscles made sore from exercise. Good to add to a spray bottle to use for cleaning benches, ovens and bathrooms.

Rosemary Oil: It is a mental stimulant used in an oil burner, great rubbed on for muscle recovery and strains, as an antiseptic, arthritis, memory enhancer, fatigue fighter, for rheumatism, headaches, coughs, flu and diabetes. Can be applied topically or used in an oil burner. Also good to add to a spray bottle to use for cleaning benches, ovens and bathrooms.

Neem Oil: From the Indian neem tree. It is very bitter with a garlic/sulfur smell. Neem oil is an excellent moisturizing oil and contains various compounds that have insecticidal and medicinal properties. It is used in making shampoos, toothpaste, soaps, cosmetics, mosquito repellants, creams and lotions, pet products lice pet shampoo, etc. It also contains vitamin E.

Great for treating many skin diseases like eczema, psoriasis, skin allergies etc. A fantastic insect repellent, Neem provides protection from not only mosquitoes, but also from biting flies, sand fleas and ticks and for controlling plant pests and diseases. Added to a spray bottle of water neem oil helps to control common pests like white flies, aphids, scales, mealy bugs, spider mites, locusts, thrips, and Japanese beetles, on plants. It also works as a fungicide and helps control powdery mildew and even on black spots, mealy bugs, spider mites & more. It is biodegradable and breaks down easily and quickly. Add a teaspoon to liquid hand soap for its antibacterial properties.

Sage Oil: Sage is calming to the nervous system, particularly in cases of depression, stress, insomnia and deep seated tension. It furthermore is a good tonic for the womb and female functions in general, such as painful periods, scanty menstruation and relaxation during labor, thus encouraging a less painful birth.

During menopause, sage oil can help reduce hot flushes, night sweats, palpitations, irritability, as well as headaches and dizziness. It is good for muscle pains, digestive disorders, kidney diseases and the cooling of inflammation of the skin. It can be used in blended massage oil, or diluted in the bath to assist with muscle pains, frigidity, depression, anxiety, menstrual problems, PMS, stress, nervous tension, insomnia, cramps and addiction.

In vapor therapy, sage oil can be used for nervous tension, stress, depression, anxiety, insomnia and menopause. It is particularly effective to help ease depression and create a more positive outlook on life and can also help to boost the creative side and intuition. Used in a cream or lotion, clary sage oil can be beneficial for skin problems, back pain and a stiff neck, as well as for body odors, PMS, skin problems and cramps. It is particularly good for balancing the production of sebum of the skin and to clear greasy complexions. It also helps with skin conditions like acne, boils and ulcers and cools painful muscles and joints. Clary sage oil's greatest benefit lies in its calming and sedating influence on the nerves, emotions, female functions, kidneys and digestive system.

NATURAL OILS TO ASSIST HEALING, DETOX AND STIMULATE HAIR GROWTH

These oils can be added to your shampoos and your conditioners, as directed.

Olive Oil Hair Wrap: Warm olive oil to tepid temperature. Apply to scalp thoroughly covering all areas and then wrap in a warm towel. This is very soothing and helps to calm and inhibit fungal growth.

Olive leaf extract is one of those super antioxidants that help with a variety of health issues and is being hailed as an awesome immune booster. With all sorts of new varieties of flu's such as swine flu having a bottle of this in the house will hopefully protect the family.

Oils To Relieve Itching: Lavender, German Chamomile and Eucalyptus Oils (Mixed together and dabbed locally on effected areas has a soothing effect). I personally recommend BE Vital by Balanced Essentials above.

Neem oil is also a very good dandruff preventative which can be added to any of the formulas detailed below and is excellent for psoriasis and eczema...I highly recommend Naturally Ngaromas' pet soap (yes it is great for humans too and gentle enough to use as a shampoo as well as the body with it's high content of Neem oil)

Oils To Assist Liver Detoxification: German or Roman Chamomile, Lavender, Geranium, Myrrh, Calendula, Frankinsense, Neroli and Rose

Oils To Stimulate Hair Growth: Rosemary, Hissop, Neroli, Lavender

Oils for Alopecia or Thinning Hair: Thyme oil, Rosemary oil and Lavender oil and Eucalyptus for stimulation

Oils For Dry Scalp: Jojoba, Neem, Evening Primrose

Recipe To Stimulate Scalp and Increase Hair Growth: (smells great too) 1 tsp Vodka, 3drops Rosemary oil, 5 drops Lavender oil. Mix and add to 1 tablespoon of water. Massage into scalp with finger tips

Alopecia Recipe: Add 12 drops jojoba oil, 6 drops Carrot oil, 6 drops Rosemary oil and 10 drops of Lavender oil to your shampoo.

Liver Detox Formula: Mix 5 drops German Chamomile, 5 drops Lavender, 2 drops Frankinsense, 2 drops Calendula and 5 drops of Rose oil to 3 oz of Almond oil. Use as a massage oil or moisturizer.

Other Dandruff Treatments:

For split ends comb in a mixture of warmed castor oil mixed with olive oil into your hair. Wrap with a towel, leave in place for half an hour. Shampoo with an added egg yolk. Add half a cup of apple cider vinegar to a gallon of cool water. Rinse with clear water to remove all traces of previous substances.

HOME REMEDIES FOR SCALP, HAIR & SKIN

http://www.dryitchyscalpremedies.com/remedy_calculator.html

CLARIFYING REMEDY TO REMOVE SHAMPOO BUILDUP

Juice of one lemon added to approx 2 tablepoons of conditioner. Mix together well and apply to wet hair making from the scalp and combing through to the ends of your hair.

LAVENDER SPRITZ (FOR REVIVING YOUR HAIR)

This is a tip I learned from Lorraine Masseys book Curly Girl –the best book I have found on how to care for wavy to curly or African american hair getting the most out of your locks. I highly recommend it!

MIX: ½ a gallon of water, 5 drops of pure lavender essential oil and 3 empty spray bottles.

You can use it throughout the day to relief a hot scalp and to give your hair a boost (or tame on humid days).

RECIPE FOR THINNING HAIR

If your hair is thinning, try increasing you intake of foods high in sulfur. Cabbage, Brussels sprouts, turnips, cauliflower as well as raspberries and cranberries are all high in sulfur. Supplement your diet with foods high in the B vitamins. Give your hair holding power with flat beer. The smell goes away in a day or so.

WALNUT RINGWORM BUSTER

This is a great ringworm recipe as well as for other fungal problems. Crush about 10 unripe walnuts and soak them in 4 cups water then boil for 15 minutes. Allow to cool and then apply liquid to effected areas. It may tingle a little which is quite normal as is slight staining of the areas (which is why walnuts also make a great hair dye).

CHAPARRAL DANDRUFF CURE

Boil 3 cups of either wine or whiskey to a boil (in a stainless steel, Silverstone or enamel - not aluminum pan) and add 1/3 cup dried chaparral (which you can buy from health stores). Simmer on low heat for 20 minutes and then steep for about 9 hours.

Massage into your scalp after washing your hair and leave to dry without rinsing.

(Note: Pouring a can of beer over your head is also helpful in treating dandruff - the hops which beer is made of has been used for centuries for medicinal purposes).

BAY LAUREL LEAF ANTI-DANDRUFF TINCTURE

Boil two cups of water then remove from heat. Add 1 ½ tablespoons of bay leaves crushed. Allow to steep for about ½ and hour then strain.

After washing hair, massage mixture into scalp and leave for about an hour before rinsing off.

PSORIASIS ECZEMA AND ACNE REMEDY

Birch is another gift from nature that native Americans used to clear up skin irritations and can be used effectively for modern problems such as psoriasis, eczema etc. Boil the bark of birch trees in water. Strain the mixture and after cooling, then apply to help clear up problems.

PSORIASIS AVOCADO TREATMENT

Put ½ cup of chamomile tea in a blender and while the blender is on slowly drizzle in 3 tablespoons of avocado oil. Blend until smooth to your psoriasis scales with a cotton ball.

BURDOCK ROOT TEA FOR ECZEMA, PSORIASIS AND SORES

Burdock root tea is excellent to aid in blood purification and detoxification. For this reason it is excellent to help clear up psoriasis and eczema and sores from the inside out.

Bring one quart (1 l) of water to the boil. Add 4 tsp dried burdock root. Cover and simmer for 10 minutes. Cool and drink preferably a couple of cups of this tea a day on an empty stomach.

SLIPPERY ELM AND ECZEMA

Add 1 Tablespoon olive oil, + 5 heaped Tablespoons of Slippery Elm bark and 5 Tablespoons of Chaparral to enough water to make a paste when slowly heated over the stove. Apply to effected areas and leave on for around half an hour then wash off.

Note: Some of these foods listed here may seem contradictory to the Psoriasis diet list. The Psoriasis list is only to be followed while you are doing a liver detox to get rid of the waste and toxic buildup in your liver. After the psoriasis has been dealt with, then you can slowly resume a normal diet.

However many people find after detoxing that their body has a natural aversion to foods that are not good for you - you may find you do not "feel like" eating them anymore and it becomes easy to stay away from them.

Habits form over time and sometimes we don't even know they are habits, especially since you have been doing them for so long. Take the time to really note what you are doing in life that is both good and bad for you. Reflection is a great way to develop another good habit and make a real lifestyle change.

Calcium: cheese, nuts, eggs, milk, yogurt, sardines, root vegetables. Coconut water Consumed 2 – 3 times a week, it is good for your skin, digestive system and is fantastic for your hair.

Essential fatty acids -- especially omega-3 fatty acids -- play a key role in skin, hair, and nails. Foods containing these acids are: Salmon, mackerel, tuna, and other oily fish. Flaxseed oil, walnuts and almonds are also a good source of these omega-3 fatty acids.

It is widely believed that omega 3 promotes brain function and studies have shown some children with concentration problems benefit hugely from taking omega 3 supplements.

Fruits and veggies will help you get folic acid as well particularly tomatoes, oranges, lemons, limes and other citrus. Eating whole and fortified grain products is good as well as beans, and lentils. B-12 is also found in high concentrations in meat, poultry, fish, and dairy products.

Once again B12 supplements can help with anxiety and stress and with all the problems we are faced with in the modern world then having knowledge about such things can only help.

Iodine: in seafood, dried kelp, iodized salt .

Iron: spinach, cockles, liver, kidneys, pulses, lentils, beans, peas, dried fruit.

Magnesium and zinc trace minerals also affect hair, so it is beneficial to take a daily multivitamin. People who lack copper can find gray hair creeping in early.

Protein is essentially what hair is made up of in the form of Keratin. Many legumes such as beans and vegetables are high in protein content. Lean meat like fish, chicken, eggs, and soy products are good sources of protein also.

Meat, fish, poultry, milk, eggs, cheese, yogurt, sunflower seeds.

Sulfur: eggs, meat, cheese, diary products .

Vitamin A: Butter, eggs, milk, carrots, tomatoes, oily fish, dark green leafy vegetables, apricots.

Vitamin B: Milk, eggs, wholegrain cereals, bread, wheat germs, nuts, soy beans and tofu, poultry, fish, meat.

Vitamin C: Blackcurrant, green peppers, citrus fruits, bananas, avocados, artichokes, leafy green vegetables.

Vitamin D: Sunlight, fish liver oils, oily fish, milk and eggs.

Vitamin E: Wheat germ, peanuts, vegetable oils, pulses, green leafy vegetables.

Vitamins B-6, B-12, and folic acid are also important to your hair. Good sources of vitamin B-6 include bananas, potatoes and spinach.

There are some amazing healthy living good books that not only have some great recipes but excite and inspire. Eating is one of life's great pleasures but when you eat something that is good for you it tastes even better. I have a great healing food cook book I got years ago from Dorling Kindersley in London which I have turned to in times of need and I found the best salsa recipe ever!

Just look at how chefs are just so popular when they start using healthier products, such as Jamie Oliver by introducing healthier meals into UK schools or Hugh Fernley-Whitingstall who cooks up the most wonderful meals from food straight off his farm or surrounding farms.

1. To stop the cycle, choose your shampoos carefully, to ensure you are not irritating your scalp or damaging it further with toxic ingredients. Invest in & use good hair care products that nourish your hair … the ones I have listed are very moisturizing and cost me far less than salon ones that dry my hair and make me itch…try some and you will see a difference.

2. Do a detox if possible – remember it does not have to be an excruciatingly tedious detox to help your body eliminate anything that is disturbing your body's natural mechanism for healing and balancing itself. However I will add that most people who do a full detox report feel light both in body and spirit. They sleep so much better, their perception sharpens after the process and levels of energy soar which also helps your body eliminate waste that's been gathering for years. SO it's worth considering – but at the very least you can take note of the "good foods" and which ones to reduce or eliminate.

3. Use the remedies to help you heal and nourish your scalp so it can repair the damage to your scalp and hair follicles. Remember, oils such as Lavender are excellent for follicle repair and stimulation whilst nourishing your scalp.

4. Eat foods high in the vitamins above. If you can introduce these to your diet or increase your intake of them…this will also aid your body in rebalancing itself and give you energy too. Being stressed is detrimental to the skin and healing process so vitamins (especially B) can make a positive impact on your skin.

5. Be kind to yourself, give yourself permission to look after you - you deserve it. Find ways to nurture/de-stress yourself such as

walking on green grass or sand without shoes on, treat yourself to a hot bath of epsom salts once a week, or sit with your eyes closed and take 10 long breaths in and out for 5 minutes just prior to rising in the morning. It's amazing the improvement to our health ad wellbeing when we can enjoy when we take time to nurture ourselves. Remember if we don't treat ourselves how can we expect others to treat us any better?

6. Try and take a more holistic approach to your health and wellbeing. When everything is well balanced and in tune you will start to feel the benefits of feeling fitter, healthier and your entire body, including your hair and scalp will change for the better.

Personal Remedy Calculator:

http://www.dryitchyscalpremedies.com/remedy_calculator.html

HAIR DYES

Here is a list of hair dyes that are mild to your scalp followed by natural remedies that with time will color your hair when used on a regular basis:

- Clairol Loving Care Color Lotion

- Igora Botanic

- Logona Henna

- Rainbow Research Henna

- Salon Formula Sun In

- Naturstyle Hair Colors

- Clairol Light Effects

BOOKS TO USE

"The Safe Shopper's Bible: A Consumer's Guide to Nontoxic Household Products" - David Steinman and Dr. Samuel Epstein

This is a fantastic book covering non-toxic household goods from food to cosmetics. I will cover some good alternatives for you in this book so it's easy to make changes and treat yourself to non-toxic, nourishing products and remedies.

PRODUCT RECOMMENDATIONS

Soothing Scalp Remedy 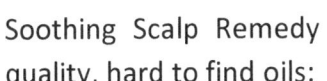 Made with the most potent, highest quality, hard to find oils:

All the best oils from this eBook in one remedy

This blend is perfect for eliminating: scalp psoriasis, scalp eczema, dandruff bacteria, burning red itchy scalp,(calms and soothes fast), head lice & will moisturize: dry scalp, brittle damaged hair. http://www.dryitchyscalpremedies.com/store

BE ESSENTIALS (NATURAL AROMATHERAPY PRODUCTS)

http://www.aroma.com.au/

Balanced Essentials supports a balanced approach to health and lifestyle as the key for a successful and happy existence.

Cheryl Gilbert is the owner/creator of Balanced Essentials and has a background in traditional medical care. With this in mind, Cheryl developed a range of aromatherapy blends, perfumes, incense and aftershave made from pure essential oils, which are energized using crystals. These products were created with the express purpose of enhancing awareness and activating self-healing.

They combine pure essential oils of the highest therapeutic quality. Each oil is subjected to quality control procedures to ensure scientific evidence of its properties. This unique collection of products, superbly presented, is created using blends of essential oils that describe the effect and are color coded to relate to an energy centre of the body. The inclusion of crystals to promote and amplify the properties of the products supports results that offer a profound and beneficial approach to health and wellbeing.

(BE Vital is excellent for application to lumps, bumps and itchy areas)

THE [A'KIN] RANGE (BY THE PURIST COMPANY)

http://www.puristusa.com/

Asia Pacific http://www.purist.com.au/

The (A'kin) difference lies in its uniquely high concentration of special nourishing and other active botanical ingredients - using only those scientifically proven to be of most benefit to the hair, skin and scalp. The result: naturally exquisitely fragranced, genuinely natural, ingredient-rich products for radiantly healthy skin and hair.

The Purist Pledge: "Each and every high quality, genuinely natural ingredient selected for [Alchemy] is present in an amount sufficient to have a significant positive effect, and is free from objectionable impurities and toxic preservatives." Will Evans Director of Research Founder - The Purist Company

- Shampoo: Most shampoos function from the action of one or two chemical cleansers and foam booster. These simple mixtures are too harsh, and consequently chemical coating agents (usually silica based) are added to counteract the stripping effect and to give the hair shine. [A'kin] takes a totally different approach. They use a synergistic complex of up to six special gentle cleansers, all derived from natural ingredients such as corn, sugar cane, palm and coconut oils and tapioca. Synthetic coating agents are not required and the hair and scalp are left naturally clean and in perfect condition to adsorb the deeply penetrating nourishing ingredients from state of the art "skin friendly" conditioners.

- Skincare: [A'kins]'s uniquely pure skincare formulations are rapidly absorbed, delivering natural nutrients deep into the skin, without the risk of irritation or allergy. Enjoy the luxury of [Alchemy]'s ingredient-rich products as they nourish and nurture your skin, while the delicate aromatherapy fragrances relax your body and soothe your soul.

OJON NUT OIL RESTORATIVE TREATMENT

http://www.ojonhaircare.com/products/OJT0001

Highly concentrated pure Ojon Nut Oil, it instantly hydrates and rebuilds distressed hair, leaving it extraordinarily soft, shiny and healthy looking. This is ideal for hair that is damaged, dry, dull or chemically treated. And these products provide essential conditioning for ALL HAIR TYPES, even if your hair is already in good condition.

SULFUR

Sulfur is very beneficial for scalp conditions, and rumor has it that it is also good for stimulating hair growth. Applied topically to the skin, sulfur-rich creams are very successful in clearing up scalp conditions, particularly in treating Seborrhoeic Dermatitis. Sulfur creams have been shown to reduce the increased sebum production, while ridding the scalp of itchy scales.

Sulfur rich foods you can supplement your diet with include eggs, seafood, beef, veal, tongue, liver, chicken, dried apricots and peaches, cabbage, Brazil nuts, peanuts and cheddar cheese. Onions, garlic and leeks are also rich in Sulfur.

SOME OTHER SPECIFIC 'SAFE' SHAMPOO BRANDS THAT CONTAIN LOW OR NO IRRITANTS

- Aveda www.aveda.com

- Mukti Botanicals

- Aubrey Organic Hair Products www.aubrey-organics.com

- Bindi Hair Wash

- Earth Science

- Faith In Nature www.faithinnature.co.uk

- Miessence   www.miessence.com

- Head Pure and Basic Lite Shampoo

- Natural Instinct   www.naturalinstinct.co.nz

- Ivory

- Jhirmack Lite

- Legona www.legona.com

- Mera

- Naturalbodycare   www.naturalbodycare-nz.com

- Paul Jenders www.pauljenders.com

- Thursday Plantation www.thursdayplantation.com

- Desert Essence Tea Tree Oil Shampoo www.desertessence.com

- Urtekram

- Ecco Bella

- Hemp seed shampoos (such as Richmond Nature brand available from health stores). Hemp is known to be very beneficial for clearing up skin irritations and soothing itching - particularly beneficial for psoriasis sufferers

- Hemp shampoos available from your local health store or online, you can also add beneficial healing oils - particularly good for psoriasis and eczema.

This concludes my e-book, "Beautiful Hair and Healthy Scalp Secrets & Remedies". I sincerely hope that you have enjoyed reading it and that you have already started making some changes. (Have fun mixing and adding).

If you apply what you now know and make conscious product choices, you will be amazed at the impact this can have on your hair and scalp. If you have any questions or feedback I would love to hear from you. I always welcome your thoughts and contribution – as it helps me to serve you best.

I feel privileged to have had the opportunity to share with you what I know. I wish you well on your journey.

If you would like to leave comments or feedback I would love to hear from you at http://www.dryitchyscalpremedies.com/contact/

www.ingramcontent.com/pod-product-compliance
Lightning Source LLC
Chambersburg PA
CBHW060638290526
45793CB00001B/306